AIR FRYER RECIPES 2021

SIDE DISH AND APPETIZER RECIPES

DELICIOUS RECIPES FOR BEGINNERS

JENNIFER WILSON

Table of Contents

Introduction

Are you always looking for easier and more modern ways to cook the best meals for you and all your loved ones?
Are you constantly searching for useful kitchen appliances that will make your work in the kitchen more fun?
Well, you don't need to search anymore! We present to you today the best kitchen appliance available these days on the market: the air fryer!

Air fryers are simply the best kitchen tools for so many reasons. Are you interested in discovering more about air fryers? Then, pay attention next!

First of all, you need to know that air fryers are special and revolutionary kitchen appliances that cook your food using the circulation of hot air. These tools use a special technology called rapid air technology. Therefore, all the food you cook in these fryers is succulent on the inside and perfectly cooked on the outside.

The next thing you need to find out about air fryers is that they allow you to cook, bake, steam and roast pretty much everything you can imagine.

Last but not least, you should know that air fryers help you cook your meals in a much healthier way.
So many people all over the world just fell in love with this great and amazing tool and now it's your turn to become one of them.

So...long story short, we recommend you to purchase an air fryer right away and to get your hands on this cooking journal as soon as possible!

We can assure you that all the meals you cook in your air fryer will taste so good and that everyone will admire your cooking skills from now one!

So, let's get started!
Have fun cooking with your great air fryer!

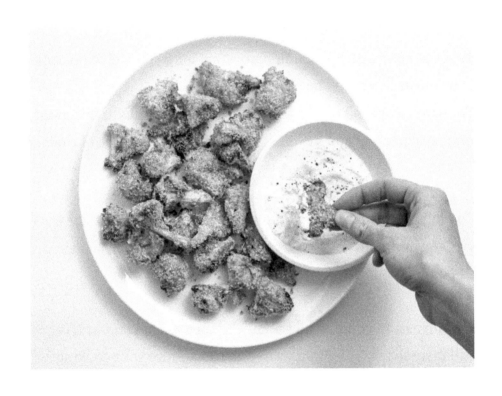

Air Fryer Side Dish and Appetizer Recipes

Zucchini Fries

Preparation time: 10 minutes **Cooking time:** 12 minutes
Servings: 4

Ingredients:

- 1 zucchini, cut into medium sticks
- A drizzle of olive oil
- Salt and black pepper to the taste
- 2 eggs, whisked
- 1 cup bread crumbs
- ½ cup flour

Directions:

1. Put flour in a bowl and mix with salt and pepper and stir.
2. Put breadcrumbs in another bowl.
3. In a third bowl mix eggs with a pinch of salt and pepper.
4. Dredge zucchini fries in flour, then in eggs and in bread crumbs at the end.

5. Grease your air fryer with some olive oil, heat up at 400 degrees F, add zucchini fries and cook them for 12 minutes.
6. Serve them as a side dish.

Enjoy!

Nutrition: calories 172, fat 3, fiber 3, carbs 7, protein 3

Herbed Tomatoes

Preparation time: 10 minutes **Cooking time:** 15 minutes

Servings: 4

Ingredients:

- 4 big tomatoes, halved and insides scooped out
- Salt and black pepper to the taste
- 1 tablespoon olive oil
- 2 garlic cloves, minced
- ½ teaspoon thyme, chopped

Directions:

1. In your air fryer, mix tomatoes with salt, pepper, oil, garlic and thyme, toss and cook at 390 degrees F for 15 minutes.
2. Divide among plates and serve them as a side dish.

Enjoy!

Nutrition: calories 112, fat 1, fiber 3, carbs 4, protein 4

Roasted Peppers

Preparation time: 10 minutes **Cooking time:** 20 minutes
Servings: 4

Ingredients:

- 1 tablespoon sweet paprika
- 1 tablespoon olive oil
- 4 red bell peppers, cut into medium strips
- 4 green bell peppers, cut into medium strips
- 4 yellow bell peppers, cut into medium strips
- 1 yellow onion, chopped
- Salt and black pepper to the taste

Directions:

1. In your air fryer, mix red bell peppers with green and yellow ones.
2. Add paprika, oil, onion, salt and pepper, toss and cook at 350 degrees F for 20 minutes.
3. Divide among plates and serve as a side dish.

Enjoy!

Nutrition: calories 142, fat 4, fiber 4, carbs 7, protein 4

Creamy Endives

Preparation time: 10 minutes **Cooking time:** 10 minutes
Servings: 6

Ingredients:

- 6 endives, trimmed and halved
- 1 teaspoon garlic powder
- ½ cup Greek yogurt
- ½ teaspoon curry powder
- Salt and black pepper to the taste
- 3 tablespoons lemon juice

Directions:

1. In a bowl, mix endives with garlic powder, yogurt, curry powder, salt, pepper and lemon juice, toss, leave aside for 10 minutes and transfer to your preheated air fryer at 350 degrees F.
2. Cook endives for 10 minutes, divide them on plates and serve as a side dish.

Enjoy!

Nutrition: calories 100, fat 2, fiber 2, carbs 7, protein 4

Delicious Roasted Carrots

Preparation time: 10 minutes **Cooking time:** 20 minutes

Servings: 4

Ingredients:

- 1 pound baby carrots
- 2 teaspoons olive oil
- 1 teaspoon herbs de Provence
- 4 tablespoons orange juice

Directions:

1. In your air fryer's basket, mix carrots with herbs de Provence, oil and orange juice, toss and cook at 320 degrees F for 20 minutes.
2. Divide among plates and serve as a side dish.

Enjoy!

Nutrition: calories 112, fat 2, fiber 3, carbs 4, protein 3

Vermouth Mushrooms

Preparation time: 10 minutes **Cooking time:** 25 minutes
Servings: 4

Ingredients:

- 1 tablespoon olive oil
- 2 pounds white mushrooms
- 2 tablespoons white vermouth
- 2 teaspoons herbs de Provence
- 2 garlic cloves, minced

Directions:

1. In your air fryer, mix oil with mushrooms, herbs de Provence and garlic, toss and cook at 350 degrees F for 20 minutes.
2. Add vermouth, toss and cook for 5 minutes more.
3. Divide among plates and serve as a side dish.

Enjoy!

Nutrition: calories 121, fat 2, fiber 5, carbs 7, protein 4

Roasted Parsnips

Preparation time: 10 minutes **Cooking time:** 40 minutes

Servings: 6

Ingredients:

- 2 pounds parsnips, peeled and cut into medium chunks
- 2 tablespoons maple syrup
- 1 tablespoon parsley flakes, dried
- 1 tablespoon olive oil

Directions:

1. Preheat your air fryer at 360 degrees F, add oil and heat it up as well.
2. Add parsnips, parsley flakes and maple syrup, toss and cook them for 40 minutes.
3. Divide among plates and serve as a side dish.

Enjoy!

Nutrition: calories 124, fat 3, fiber 3, carbs 7, protein 4

Barley Risotto

Preparation time: 10 minutes **Cooking time:** 30 minutes
Servings: 8

Ingredients:

- 5 cups veggie stock
- 3 tablespoons olive oil
- 2 yellow onions, chopped
- 2 garlic cloves, minced
- ¾ pound barley
- 3 ounces mushrooms, sliced
- 2 ounces skim milk
- 1 teaspoon thyme, dried
- 1 teaspoon tarragon, dried
- Salt and black pepper to the taste
- 2 pounds sweet potato, peeled and chopped

Directions:

1. Put stock in a pot, add barley, stir, bring to a boil over medium heat and cook for 15 minutes.
2. Heat up your air fryer at 350 degrees F, add oil and heat it up.

3. Add barley, onions, garlic, mushrooms, milk, salt, pepper, tarragon and sweet potato, stir and cook for 15 minutes more.

4. Divide among plates and serve as a side dish.

Enjoy!

Nutrition: calories 124, fat 4, fiber 4, carbs 6, protein 4

Glazed Beets

Preparation time: 10 minutes **Cooking time:** 40 minutes
Servings: 8

Ingredients:

- 3 pounds small beets, trimmed
- 4 tablespoons maple syrup
- 1 tablespoon duck fat

Directions:

1. Heat up your air fryer at 360 degrees F, add duck fat and heat it up.
2. Add beets and maple syrup, toss and cook for 40 minutes.
3. Divide among plates and serve as a side dish.

Enjoy!

Nutrition: calories 121, fat 3, fiber 2, carbs 3, protein 4

Beer Risotto

Preparation time: 10 minutes **Cooking time:** 30 minutes
Servings: 4

Ingredients:
- 2 tablespoons olive oil
- 2 yellow onions, chopped
- 1 cup mushrooms, sliced
- 1 teaspoon basil, dried
- 1 teaspoon oregano, dried
- 1 and ½ cups rice
- 2 cups beer
- 2 cups chicken stock
- 1 tablespoon butter
- ½ cup parmesan, grated

Directions:

1. In a dish that fits your air fryer, mix oil with onions, mushrooms, basil and oregano and stir.
2. Add rice, beer, butter, stock and butter, stir again, place in your air fryer's basket and cook at 350 degrees F for 30 minutes.
3. Divide among plates and serve with grated parmesan on top as a side dish.

Enjoy!

Nutrition: calories 142, fat 4, fiber 4, carbs 6, protein 4

Cauliflower Rice

Preparation time: 10 minutes **Cooking time:** 40 minutes
Servings: 8

Ingredients:

- 1 tablespoon peanut oil
- 1 tablespoon sesame oil
- 4 tablespoons soy sauce
- 3 garlic cloves, minced
- 1 tablespoon ginger, grated
- Juice from ½ lemon
- 1 cauliflower head, riced
- 9 ounces water chestnuts, drained
- ¾ cup peas
- 15 ounces mushrooms, chopped
- 1 egg, whisked

Directions:

1. In your air fryer, mix cauliflower rice with peanut oil, sesame oil, soy sauce, garlic, ginger and lemon juice, stir, cover and cook at 350 degrees F for 20 minutes.
2. Add chestnuts, peas, mushrooms and egg, toss and cook at 360 degrees F for 20 minutes more.
3. Divide among plates and serve for breakfast.

Enjoy!

Nutrition: calories 142, fat 3, fiber 2, carbs 6, protein 4

Carrots and Rhubarb

Preparation time: 10 minutes **Cooking time:** 40 minutes

Servings: 4

Ingredients:

- 1 pound baby carrots
- 2 teaspoons walnut oil
- 1 pound rhubarb, roughly chopped
- 1 orange, peeled, cut into medium segments and zest grated
- ½ cup walnuts, halved
- ½ teaspoon stevia

Directions:

1. Put the oil in your air fryer, add carrots, toss and fry them at 380 degrees F for 20 minutes.
2. Add rhubarb, orange zest, stevia and walnuts, toss and cook for 20 minutes more.
3. Add orange segments, toss and serve as a side dish.

Enjoy!

Nutrition: calories 172, fat 2, fiber 3, carbs 4, protein 4

Roasted Eggplant

Preparation time: 10 minutes **Cooking time:** 20 minutes

Servings: 6

Ingredients:

- 1 and ½ pounds eggplant, cubed
- 1 tablespoon olive oil
- 1 teaspoon garlic powder
- 1 teaspoon onion powder
- 1 teaspoon sumac
- 2 teaspoons za'atar
- Juice from ½ lemon
- 2 bay leaves

Directions:

1. In your air fryer, mix eggplant cubes with oil, garlic powder, onion powder, sumac, za'atar, lemon juice and bay leaves, toss and cook at 370 degrees F for 20 minutes.
2. Divide among plates and serve as a side dish.

Enjoy!

Nutrition: calories 172, fat 4, fiber 7, carbs 12, protein 3

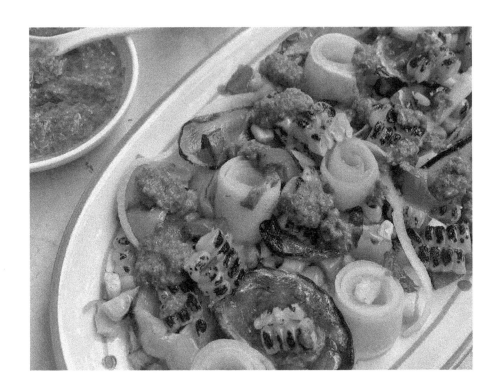

Delicious Air Fried Broccoli

Preparation time: 10 minutes **Cooking time:** 20 minutes

Servings: 4

Ingredients:

- 1 tablespoon duck fat
- 1 broccoli head, florets separated
- 3 garlic cloves, minced
- Juice from ½ lemon
- 1 tablespoon sesame seeds

Directions:

1. Heat up your air fryer at 350 degrees F, add duck fat and heat as well.
2. Add broccoli, garlic, lemon juice and sesame seeds, toss and cook for 20 minutes.
3. Divide among plates and serve as a side dish.

Enjoy!

Nutrition: calories 132, fat 3, fiber 3, carbs 6, protein 4

Onion Rings Side Dish

Preparation time: 10 minutes **Cooking time:** 10 minutes
Servings: 3

Ingredients:

- 1 onion cut into medium slices and rings separated
- 1 and ¼ cups white flour
- A pinch of salt
- 1 egg
- 1 cup milk
- 1 teaspoon baking powder
- ¾ cup bread crumbs

Directions:

1. In a bowl, mix flour with salt and baking powder, stir, dredge onion rings in this mix and place them on a separate plate.
2. Add milk and egg to flour mix and whisk well.
3. Dip onion rings in this mix, dredge them in breadcrumbs, put them in your air fryer's basket and cook them at 360 degrees F for 10 minutes.
4. Divide among plates and serve as a side dish for a steak.

Enjoy!

Nutrition: calories 140, fat 8, fiber 20, carbs 12, protein 3

Rice and Sausage Side Dish

Preparation time: 10 minutes **Cooking time:** 20 minutes

Servings: 4

Ingredients:

- 2 cups white rice, already boiled
- 1 tablespoon butter
- Salt and black pepper to the taste
- 4 garlic cloves, minced
- 1 pork sausage, chopped
- 2 tablespoons carrot, chopped
- 3 tablespoons cheddar cheese, grated
- 2 tablespoons mozzarella cheese, shredded

Directions:

1. Heat up your air fryer at 350 degrees F, add butter, melt it, add garlic, stir and brown for 2 minutes.
2. Add sausage, salt, pepper, carrots and rice, stir and cook at 350 degrees F for 10 minutes.
3. Add cheddar and mozzarella, toss, divide among plates and serve as a side dish.

Enjoy!

Nutrition: calories 240, fat 12, fiber 5, carbs 20, protein 13

Potatoes Patties

Preparation time: 10 minutes **Cooking time:** 8 minutes

Servings: 4

Ingredients:

- 4 potatoes, cubed, boiled and mashed
- 1 cup parmesan, grated
- Salt and black pepper to the taste
- A pinch of nutmeg
- 2 egg yolks
- 2 tablespoons white flour
- 3 tablespoons chives, chopped

For the breading:

- ¼ cup white flour
- 3 tablespoons vegetable oil
- 2 eggs, whisked
- ¼ cup bread crumbs

Directions:

1. In a bowl, mix mashed potatoes with egg yolks, salt, pepper, nutmeg, parmesan, chives and 2 tablespoons

flour, stir well, shape medium cakes and place them on a plate.

2. In another bowl, mix vegetable oil with bread crumbs and stir,.

3. Put whisked eggs in a third bowl and ¼ cup flour in a forth one.

4. Dip cakes in flour, then in eggs and in breadcrumbs at the end, place them in your air fryer's basket, cook them at 390 degrees F for 8 minutes, divide among plates and serve as a side dish.

Enjoy!

Nutrition: calories 140, fat 3, fiber 4, carbs 17, protein 4

Simple Potato Chips

Preparation time: 30 minutes **Cooking time:** 30 minutes
Servings: 4

Ingredients:

- 4 potatoes, scrubbed, peeled into thin chips, soaked in water for 30 minutes, drained and pat dried
- Salt the taste
- 1 tablespoon olive oil
- 2 teaspoons rosemary, chopped

Directions:

1. In a bowl, mix potato chips with salt and oil toss to coat, place them in your air fryer's basket and cook at 330 degrees F for 30 minutes.
2. Divide among plates, sprinkle rosemary all over and serve as a side dish.

Enjoy!

Nutrition: calories 200, fat 4, fiber 4, carbs 14, protein 5

Avocado Fries

Preparation time: 10 minutes **Cooking time:** 10 minutes
Servings: 4

Ingredients:

- 1 avocado, pitted, peeled, sliced and cut into medium fries
- Salt and black pepper to the taste
- ½ cup panko bread crumbs
- 1 tablespoon lemon juice
- 1 egg, whisked
- 1 tablespoon olive oil

Directions:

1. In a bowl, mix panko with salt and pepper and stir.
2. In another bowl, mix egg with a pinch of salt and whisk.
3. In a third bowl, mix avocado fries with lemon juice and oil and toss.
4. Dip fries in egg, then in panko, place them in your air fryer's basket and cook at 390 degrees F for 10 minutes, shaking halfway.
5. Divide among plates and serve as a side dish.

Enjoy!

Nutrition: calories 130, fat 11, fiber 3, carbs 16, protein 4

Veggie Fries

Preparation time: 10 minutes **Cooking time:** 30 minutes
Servings: 4

Ingredients:

- 4 parsnips, cut into medium sticks
- 2 sweet potatoes cut into medium sticks
- 4 mixed carrots cut into medium sticks
- Salt and black pepper to the taste
- 2 tablespoons rosemary, chopped
- 2 tablespoons olive oil
- 1 tablespoon flour
- ½ teaspoon garlic powder

Directions:

1. Put veggie fries in a bowl, add oil, garlic powder, salt, pepper, flour and rosemary and toss to coat.
2. Put sweet potatoes in your preheated air fryer, cook them for 10 minutes at 350 degrees F and transfer them to a platter.
3. Put parsnip fries in your air fryer, cook for 5 minutes and transfer over potato fries.

4. Put carrot fries in your air fryer, cook for 15 minutes at 350 degrees F and transfer to the platter with the other fries.

5. Divide veggie fries on plates and serve them as a side dish.

Enjoy!

Nutrition: calories 100, fat 0, fiber 4, carbs 7, protein 4

Air Fried Creamy Cabbage

Preparation time: 10 minutes **Cooking time:** 20 minute
Servings: 4

Ingredients:

- 1 green cabbage head, chopped
- 1 yellow onion, chopped
- Salt and black pepper to the taste
- 4 bacon slices, chopped
- 1 cup whipped cream
- 2 tablespoons cornstarch

Directions:

1. Put cabbage, bacon and onion in your air fryer.
2. In a bowl, mix cornstarch with cream, salt and pepper, stir and add over cabbage.
3. Toss, cook at 400 degrees F for 20 minutes, divide among plates and serve as a side dish.

Enjoy!

Nutrition: calories 208, fat 10, fiber 3, carbs 16, protein 5

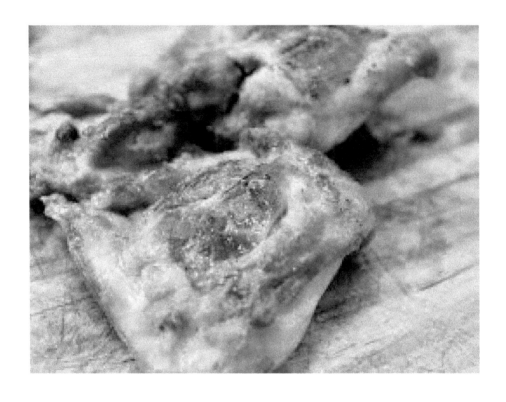

Tortilla Chips

Preparation time: 10 minutes **Cooking time:** 6 minutes

Servings: 4

Ingredients:

- 8 corn tortillas, cut into triangles
- Salt and black pepper to the taste
- 1 tablespoon olive oil
- A pinch of garlic powder
- A pinch of sweet paprika

Directions:

1. In a bowl, mix tortilla chips with oil, add salt, pepper, garlic powder and paprika, toss well, place them in your air fryer's basket and cook them at 400 degrees F for 6 minutes.
2. Serve them as a side for a fish dish.

Enjoy!

Nutrition: calories 53, fat 1, fiber 1, carbs 6, protein 4

Zucchini Croquettes

Preparation time: 10 minutes **Cooking time:** 10 minutes
Servings: 4

Ingredients:

- 1 carrot, grated
- 1 zucchini, grated
- 2 slices of bread, crumbled
- 1 egg
- Salt and black pepper to the taste
- ½ teaspoon sweet paprika
- 1 teaspoon garlic, minced
- 2 tablespoons parmesan cheese, grated
- 1 tablespoon corn flour

Directions:

1. Put zucchini in a bowl, add salt, leave aside for 10 minutes, squeeze excess water and transfer them to another bowl.
2. Add carrots, salt, pepper, paprika, garlic, flour, parmesan, egg and bread crumbs, stir well, shape 8

croquettes, place them in your air fryer and cook at 360 degrees F for 10 minutes.

3. Divide among plates and serve as a side dish

Enjoy!

Nutrition: calories 100, fat 3, fiber 1, carbs 7, protein 4

Creamy Potatoes

Preparation time: 10 minutes **Cooking time:** 20 minutes

Servings: 4

Ingredients:

- 1 an ½ pounds potatoes, peeled and cubed
- 2 tablespoons olive oil
- Salt and black pepper to the taste
- 1 tablespoon hot paprika
- 1 cup Greek yogurt

Directions:

1. Put potatoes in a bowl, add water to cover, leave aside for 10 minutes, drain, pat dry them, transfer to another bowl, add salt, pepper, paprika and half of the oil and toss them well.
2. Put potatoes in your air fryer's basket and cook at 360 degrees F for 20 minutes.
3. In a bowl, mix yogurt with salt, pepper and the rest of the oil and whisk.
4. Divide potatoes on plates, drizzle yogurt dressing all over, toss them and serve as a side dish.

Enjoy!

Nutrition: calories 170, fat 3, fiber 5, carbs 20, protein 5

Mushroom Cakes

Preparation time: 10 minutes **Cooking time:** 8 minutes **Servings:** 8

Ingredients:

- 4 ounces mushrooms, chopped
- 1 yellow onion, chopped
- Salt and black pepper to the taste
- ½ teaspoon nutmeg, ground
- 2 tablespoons olive oil
- 1 tablespoon butter
- 1 and ½ tablespoon flour
- 1 tablespoon bread crumbs
- 14 ounces milk

Directions:

1. Heat up a pan with the butter over medium high heat, add onion and mushrooms, stir, cook for 3 minutes, add flour, stir well again and take off heat.
2. Add milk gradually, salt, pepper and nutmeg, stir and leave aside to cool down completely.
3. In a bowl, mix oil with bread crumbs and whisk.

4. Take spoonfuls of the mushroom filling, add to breadcrumbs mix, coat well, shape patties out of this mix, place them in your air fryer's basket and cook at 400 degrees F for 8 minutes.
5. Divide among plates and serve as a side for a steak

Enjoy!

Nutrition: calories 192, fat 2, fiber 1, carbs 16, protein 6

Creamy Roasted Peppers Side Dish

Preparation time: 10 minutes **Cooking time:** 10 minutes
Servings: 4

Ingredients:

- 1 tablespoon lemon juice
- 1 red bell pepper
- 1 green bell pepper
- 1 yellow bell pepper
- 1 lettuce head, cut into strips
- 1 ounce rocket leaves
- Salt and black pepper to the taste
- 3 tablespoons Greek yogurt
- 2 tablespoons olive oil

Directions:

1. Place bell peppers in your air fryer's basket, cook at 400 degrees F for 10 minutes, transfer to a bowl, leave aside for 10 minutes, peel them, discard seeds, cut

them in strips, transfer to a larger bowl, add rocket leaves and lettuce strips and toss.

2. In a bowl, mix oil with lemon juice, yogurt, salt and pepper and whisk well.

3. Add this over bell peppers mix, toss to coat, divide among plates and serve as a side salad.

Enjoy!

Nutrition: calories 170, fat 1, fiber 1, carbs 2, protein 6

Greek Veggie Side Dish

Preparation time: 10 minutes **Cooking time:** 45 minutes
Servings: 4

Ingredients:

- 1 eggplant, sliced
- 1 zucchini, sliced
- 2 red bell peppers, chopped
- 2 garlic cloves, minced
- 3 tablespoons olive oil
- 1 bay leaf
- 1 thyme spring, chopped
- 2 onions, chopped
- 4 tomatoes, cut into quarters
- Salt and black pepper to the taste

Directions:

1. In your air fryer's pan, mix eggplant slices with zucchini ones, bell peppers, garlic, oil, bay leaf, thyme, onions, tomatoes, salt and pepper, toss and cook them at 300 degrees F for 35 minutes.
2. Divide among plates and serve as a side dish.

Enjoy!

Nutrition: calories 200, fat 1, fiber 3, carbs 7, protein 6

Yellow Squash and Zucchinis Side Dish

Preparation time: 10 minutes **Cooking time:** 35 minutes

Servings: 4

Ingredients:

- 6 teaspoons olive oil
- 1 pound zucchinis, sliced
- ½ pound carrots, cubed
- 1 yellow squash, halved, deseeded and cut into chunks
- Salt and white pepper to the taste
- 1 tablespoon tarragon, chopped

Directions:

1. In your air fryer's basket, mix zucchinis with carrots, squash, salt, pepper and oil, toss well and cook at 400 degrees F for 25 minutes.
2. Divide them on plates and serve as a side dish with tarragon sprinkled on top.

Enjoy!

Nutrition: calories 160, fat 2, fiber 1, carbs 5, protein 5

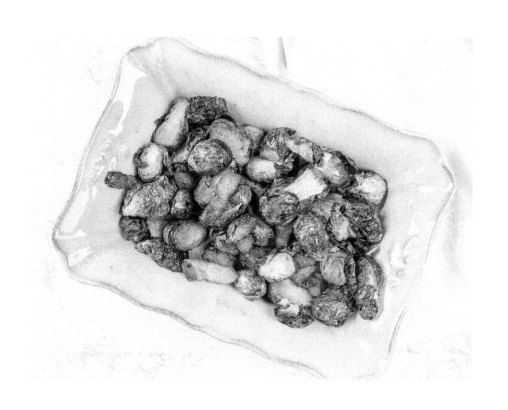

Flavored Cauliflower Side Dish

Preparation time: 10 minutes **Cooking time:** 10 minutes
Servings: 4

Ingredients:

- 12 cauliflower florets, steamed
- Salt and black pepper to the taste
- ¼ teaspoon turmeric powder
- 1 and ½ teaspoon red chili powder
- 1 tablespoon ginger, grated
- 2 teaspoons lemon juice
- 3 tablespoons white flour
- 2 tablespoons water
- Cooking spray
- ½ teaspoon corn flour

Directions:

1. In a bowl, mix chili powder with turmeric powder, ginger paste, salt, pepper, lemon juice, white flour, corn flour and water, stir, add cauliflower, toss well and transfer them to your air fryer's basket.

2. Coat them with cooking spray, cook them at 400 degrees F for 10 minutes, divide among plates and serve as a side dish.

Enjoy!

Nutrition: calories 70, fat 1, fiber 2, carbs 12, protein 3

Coconut Cream Potato es

Preparation time: 10 minutes **Cooking time:** 20 minutes

Servings: 4

Ingredients:

- 2 eggs, whisked
- Salt and black pepper to the taste
- 1 tablespoon cheddar cheese, grated
- 1 tablespoon flour
- 2 potatoes, sliced
- 4 ounces coconut cream

Directions:

1. Place potato slices in your air fryer's basket and cook at 360 degrees F for 10 minutes.
2. Meanwhile, in a bowl, mix eggs with coconut cream, salt, pepper and flour.
3. Arrange potatoes in your air fryer's pan, add coconut cream mix over them, sprinkle cheese, return to air fryer's basket and cook at 400 degrees F for 10 minutes more.
4. Divide among plates and serve as a side dish.

Enjoy!

Nutrition: calories 170, fat 4, fiber 1, carbs 15, protein 17

Cajun Onion Wedges

Preparation time: 10 minutes **Cooking time:** 15 minutes

Servings: 4

Ingredients:

- 2 big white onions, cut into wedges
- Salt and black pepper to the taste
- 2 eggs
- ¼ cup milk
- 1/3 cup panko
- A drizzle of olive oil
- 1 and ½ teaspoon paprika
- 1 teaspoon garlic powder
- ½ teaspoon Cajun seasoning

Directions:

1. In a bowl, mix panko with Cajun seasoning and oil and stir.
2. In another bowl, mix egg with milk, salt and pepper and stir.
3. Sprinkle onion wedges with paprika and garlic powder, dip them in egg mix, then in bread crumbs mix, place in

your air fryer's basket, cook at 360 degrees F for 10 minutes, flip and cook for 5 minutes more.

4. Divide among plates and serve as a side dish.

Enjoy!

Nutrition: calories 200, fat 2, fiber 2, carbs 14, protein 7

Wild Rice Pilaf

Preparation time: 10 minutes **Cooking time:** 25 minutes
Servings: 12

Ingredients:

- 1 shallot, chopped
- 1 teaspoon garlic, minced
- A drizzle of olive oil
- 1 cup farro
- ¾ cup wild rice
- 4 cups chicken stock
- Salt and black pepper to the taste
- 1 tablespoon parsley, chopped
- ½ cup hazelnuts, toasted and chopped
- ¾ cup cherries, dried
- Chopped chives for serving

Directions:

1. In a dish that fits your air fryer, mix shallot with garlic, oil, faro, wild rice, stock, salt, pepper, parsley, hazelnuts and cherries, stir, place in your air fryer's basket and cook at 350 degrees F for 25 minutes.

2. Divide among plates and serve as a side dish.

Enjoy!

Nutrition: calories 142, fat 4, fiber 4, carbs 16, protein 4

Pumpkin Rice

Preparation time: 5 minutes **Cooking time:** 30 minutes

Servings: 4

Ingredients:

- 2 tablespoons olive oil
- 1 small yellow onion, chopped
- 2 garlic cloves, minced
- 12 ounces white rice
- 4 cups chicken stock
- 6 ounces pumpkin puree
- ½ teaspoon nutmeg
- 1 teaspoon thyme, chopped
- ½ teaspoon ginger, grated
- ½ teaspoon cinnamon powder
- ½ teaspoon allspice
- 4 ounces heavy cream

Directions:

1. In a dish that fits your air fryer, mix oil with onion, garlic, rice, stock, pumpkin puree, nutmeg, thyme, ginger, cinnamon, allspice and cream, stir well, place in

your air fryer's basket and cook at 360 degrees F for 30 minutes.

2. Divide among plates and serve as a side dish.

Enjoy!

Nutrition: calories 261, fat 6, fiber 7, carbs 29, protein 4

Colored Veggie Rice

Preparation time: 10 minutes **Cooking time:** 25 minutes

Servings: 4

Ingredients:

- 2 cups basmati rice
- 1 cup mixed carrots, peas, corn and green beans
- 2 cups water
- ½ teaspoon green chili, minced
- ½ teaspoon ginger, grated
- 3 garlic cloves, minced
- 2 tablespoons butter
- 1 teaspoon cinnamon powder
- 1 tablespoon cumin seeds
- 2 bay leaves
- 3 whole cloves
- 5 black peppercorns
- 2 whole cardamoms
- 1 tablespoon sugar
- Salt to the taste

Directions:

1. Put the water in a heat proof dish that fits your air fryer, add rice, mixed veggies, green chili, grated ginger, garlic cloves, cinnamon, cloves, butter, cumin seeds, bay leaves, cardamoms, black peppercorns, salt and sugar, stir, put in your air fryer's basket and cook at 370 degrees F for 25 minutes.
2. Divide among plates and serve as a side dish.

Enjoy!

Nutrition: calories 283, fat 4, fiber 8, carbs 34, protein 14

Potato Casserole

Preparation time: 15 minutes **Cooking time:** 40 minutes
Servings: 4

Ingredients:

- 3 pounds sweet potatoes, scrubbed
- ¼ cup milk
- ½ teaspoon nutmeg, ground
- 2 tablespoons white flour
- ¼ teaspoon allspice, ground
- Salt to the taste

For the topping:

- ½ cup almond flour
- ½ cup walnuts, soaked, drained and ground
- ¼ cup pecans, soaked, drained and ground
- ¼ cup coconut, shredded
- 1 tablespoon chia seeds
- ¼ cup sugar
- 1 teaspoon cinnamon powder
- 5 tablespoons butter

Directions:

1. Place potatoes in your air fryer's basket, prick them with a fork and cook at 360 degrees F for 30 minutes.
2. Meanwhile, in a bowl, mix almond flour with pecans, walnuts, ¼ cup coconut, ¼ cup sugar, chia seeds, 1 teaspoon cinnamon and the butter and stir everything.
3. Transfer potatoes to a cutting board, cool them, peel and place them in a baking dish that fits your air fryer.
4. Add milk, flour, salt, nutmeg and allspice and stir
5. Add crumble mix you've made earlier on top, place dish in your air fryer's basket and cook at 400 degrees F for 8 minutes.
6. Divide among plates and serve as a side dish.

Enjoy!

Nutrition: calories 162, fat 4, fiber 8, carbs 18, protein 4

Lemony Artichokes

Preparation time: 10 minutes **Cooking time:** 15 minutes
Servings: 4

Ingredients:

- 2 medium artichokes, trimmed and halved
- Cooking spray
- 2 tablespoons lemon juice
- Salt and black pepper to the taste

Directions:

1. Grease your air fryer with cooking spray, add artichokes, drizzle lemon juice and sprinkle salt and black pepper and cook them at 380 degrees F for 15 minutes.
2. Divide them on plates and serve as a side dish.

Enjoy!

Nutrition: calories 121, fat 3, fiber 6, carbs 9, protein 4

Cauliflower and Broccoli Delight

Preparation time: 10 minutes **Cooking time:** 7 minutes
Servings: 4

Ingredients:

- 2 cauliflower heads, florets separated and steamed
- 1 broccoli head, florets separated and steamed
- Zest from 1 orange, grated
- Juice from 1 orange
- A pinch of hot pepper flakes
- 4 anchovies
- 1 tablespoon capers, chopped
- Salt and black pepper to the taste
- 4 tablespoons olive oil

Directions:

1. In a bowl, mix orange zest with orange juice, pepper flakes, anchovies, capers salt, pepper and olive oil and whisk well.
2. Add broccoli and cauliflower, toss well, transfer them to your air fryer's basket and cook at 400 degrees F for 7 minutes.
3. Divide among plates and serve as a side dish with some of the orange vinaigrette drizzled on top.

Enjoy!

Nutrition: calories 300, fat 4, fiber 7, carbs 28, protein 4

Garlic Beet Wedges

Preparation time: 10 minutes **Cooking time:** 15 minutes

Servings: 4

Ingredients:

- 4 beets, washed, peeled and cut into large wedges
- 1 tablespoon olive oil
- Salt and black to the taste
- 2 garlic cloves, minced
- 1 teaspoon lemon juice

Directions:

1. In a bowl, mix beets with oil, salt, pepper, garlic and lemon juice, toss well, transfer to your air fryer's basket and cook them at 400 degrees F for 15 minutes.
2. Divide beets wedges on plates and serve as a side dish.

Enjoy!

Nutrition: calories 182, fat 6, fiber 3, carbs 8, protein 2

Fried Red Cabbage

Preparation time: 10 minutes **Cooking time:** 15 minutes
Servings: 4

Ingredients:

- 4 garlic cloves, minced
- ½ cup yellow onion, chopped
- 1 tablespoon olive oil
- 6 cups red cabbage, chopped
- 1 cup veggie stock
- 1 tablespoon apple cider vinegar
- 1 cup applesauce
- Salt and black pepper to the taste

Directions:

1. In a heat proof dish that fits your air fryer, mix cabbage with onion, garlic, oil, stock, vinegar, applesauce, salt and pepper, toss really well, place dish in your air fryer's basket and cook at 380 degrees F for 15 minutes.
2. Divide among plates and serve as a side dish.

Enjoy!

Nutrition: calories 172, fat 7, fiber 7, carbs 14, protein 5

Artichokes and Tarragon Sauce

Preparation time: 10 minutes **Cooking time:** 18 minutes

Servings: 4

Ingredients:

- 4 artichokes, trimmed
- 2 tablespoons tarragon, chopped
- 2 tablespoons chicken stock
- Lemon zest from 2 lemons, grated
- 2 tablespoons lemon juice
- 1 celery stalk, chopped
- ½ cup olive oil
- Salt to the taste

Directions:

1. In your food processor, mix tarragon, chicken stock, lemon zest, lemon juice, celery, salt and olive oil and pulse very well.
2. In a bowl, mix artichokes with tarragon and lemon sauce, toss well, transfer them to your air fryer's basket and cook at 380 degrees F for 18 minutes.
3. Divide artichokes on plates, drizzle the rest of the sauce all over and serve as a side dish.

Enjoy!

Nutrition: calories 215, fat 3, fiber 8, carbs 28, protein 6

Brussels Sprouts and Pomegranate Seeds Side Dish

Preparation time: 5 minutes **Cooking time:** 10 minutes

Servings: 4

Ingredients:

- 1 pound Brussels sprouts, trimmed and halved
- Salt and black pepper to the taste
- 1 cup pomegranate seeds
- ¼ cup pine nuts, toasted
- 1 tablespoons olive oil
- 2 tablespoons veggie stock

Directions:

1. In a heat proof dish that fits your air fryer, mix Brussels sprouts with salt, pepper, pomegranate seeds, pine nuts, oil and stock, stir, place in your air fryer's basket and cook at 390 degrees F for 10 minutes.
2. Divide among plates and serve as a side dish.

Enjoy!

Nutrition: calories 152, fat 4, fiber 7, carbs 12, protein 3

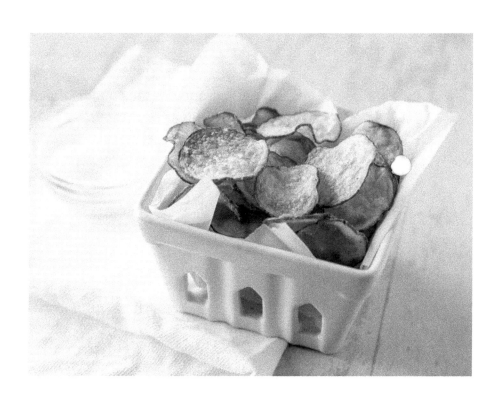

Crispy Brussels Sprouts and Potatoes

Preparation time: 10 minutes **Cooking time:** 8 minutes
Servings: 4

Ingredients:

- 1 and ½ pounds Brussels sprouts, washed and trimmed
- 1 cup new potatoes, chopped
- 1 and ½ tablespoons bread crumbs
- Salt and black pepper to the taste
- 1 and ½ tablespoons butter

Directions:

1. Put Brussels sprouts and potatoes in your air fryer's pan, add bread crumbs, salt, pepper and butter, toss well and cook at 400 degrees F for 8 minutes.
2. Divide among plates and serve as a side dish.

Enjoy!

Nutrition: calories 152, fat 3, fiber 7, carbs 17, protein 4

Coconut Chicken Bites

Preparation time: 10 minutes **Cooking time:** 13 minutes
Servings: 4

Ingredients:

- 2 teaspoons garlic powder
- 2 eggs
- Salt and black pepper to the taste
- ¾ cup panko bread crumbs
- ¾ cup coconut, shredded
- Cooking spray
- 8 chicken tenders

Directions:

1. In a bowl, mix eggs with salt, pepper and garlic powder and whisk well.
2. In another bowl, mix coconut with panko and stir well.
3. Dip chicken tenders in eggs mix and then coat in coconut one well.

4. Spray chicken bites with cooking spray, place them in your air fryer's basket and cook them at 350 degrees F for 10 minutes.

5. Arrange them on a platter and serve as an appetizer.

Enjoy!

Nutrition: calories 252, fat 4, fiber 2, carbs 14, protein 24

Buffalo Cauliflower Snack

Preparation time: 10 minutes **Cooking time:** 15 minutes

Servings: 4

Ingredients:

- 4 cups cauliflower florets
- 1 cup panko bread crumbs
- ¼ cup butter, melted
- ¼ cup buffalo sauce
- Mayonnaise for serving

Directions:

1. In a bowl, mix buffalo sauce with butter and whisk well.
2. Dip cauliflower florets in this mix and coat them in panko bread crumbs.
3. Place them in your air fryer's basket and cook at 350 degrees F for 15 minutes.
4. Arrange them on a platter and serve with mayo on the side.

Enjoy!

Nutrition: calories 241, fat 4, fiber 7, carbs 8, protein 4

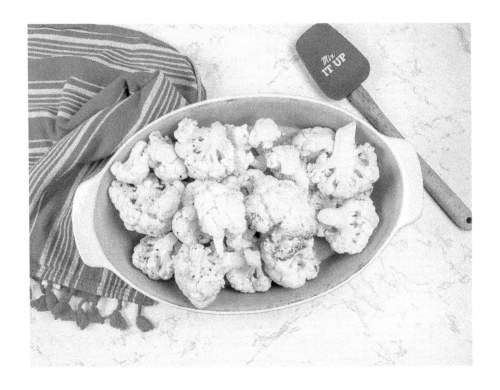

Banana Snack

Preparation time: 10 minutes **Cooking time:** 5 minutes

Servings: 8

Ingredients:

- 16 baking cups crust
- ¼ cup peanut butter
- ¾ cup chocolate chips
- 1 banana, peeled and sliced into 16 pieces
- 1 tablespoon vegetable oil

Directions:

1. Put chocolate chips in a small pot, heat up over low heat, stir until it melts and take off heat.
2. In a bowl, mix peanut butter with coconut oil and whisk well.
3. Spoon 1 teaspoon chocolate mix in a cup, add 1 banana slice and top with 1 teaspoon butter mix
4. Repeat with the rest of the cups, place them all into a dish that fits your air fryer, cook at 320 degrees F for 5 minutes, transfer to a freezer and keep there until you serve them as a snack.

Enjoy!

Nutrition: calories 70, fat 4, fiber 1, carbs 10, protein 1

Potato Spread

Preparation time: 10 minutes **Cooking time:** 10 minutes
Servings: 10

Ingredients:

- 19 ounces canned garbanzo beans, drained
- 1 cup sweet potatoes, peeled and chopped
- ¼ cup tahini
- 2 tablespoons lemon juice
- 1 tablespoon olive oil
- 5 garlic cloves, minced
- ½ teaspoon cumin, ground
- 2 tablespoons water
- A pinch of salt and white pepper

Directions:

1. Put potatoes in your air fryer's basket, cook them at 360 degrees F for 15 minutes, cool them down, peel, put them in your food processor and pulse well. basket,
2. Add sesame paste, garlic, beans, lemon juice, cumin, water and oil and pulse really well.
3. Add salt and pepper, pulse again, divide into bowls and serve.

Enjoy!

Nutrition: calories 200, fat 3, fiber 10, carbs 20, protein 11

Mexican Apple Snack

Preparation time: 10 minutes **Cooking time:** 5 minutes

Servings: 4

Ingredients:

- 3 big apples, cored, peeled and cubed
- 2 teaspoons lemon juice
- ¼ cup pecans, chopped
- ½ cup dark chocolate chips
- ½ cup clean caramel sauce

Directions:

1. In a bowl, mix apples with lemon juice, stir and transfer to a pan that fits your air fryer.
2. Add chocolate chips, pecans, drizzle the caramel sauce, toss, introduce in your air fryer and cook at 320 degrees F for 5 minutes.
3. Toss gently, divide into small bowls and serve right away as a snack.

Enjoy!

Nutrition: calories 200, fat 4, fiber 3, carbs 20, protein 3

Shrimp Muffins

Preparation time: 10 minutes **Cooking time:** 26 minutes
Servings: 6

Ingredients:
- 1 spaghetti squash, peeled and halved
- 2 tablespoons mayonnaise
- 1 cup mozzarella, shredded
- 8 ounces shrimp, peeled, cooked and chopped
- 1 and ½ cups panko
- 1 teaspoon parsley flakes
- 1 garlic clove, minced
- Salt and black pepper to the taste
- Cooking spray

Directions:
1. Put squash halves in your air fryer, cook at 350 degrees F for 16 minutes, leave aside to cool down and scrape flesh into a bowl.
2. Add salt, pepper, parsley flakes, panko, shrimp, mayo and mozzarella and stir well.

3. Spray a muffin tray that fits your air fryer with cooking spray and divide squash and shrimp mix in each cup.

4. Introduce in the fryer and cook at 360 degrees F for 10 minutes.

5. Arrange muffins on a platter and serve as a snack.

Enjoy!

Nutrition: calories 60, fat 2, fiber 0.4, carbs 4, protein 4

Zucchini Cakes

Preparation time: 10 minutes **Cooking time:** 12 minutes
Servings: 12

Ingredients:

- Cooking spray
- ½ cup dill, chopped
- 1 egg
- ½ cup whole wheat flour
- Salt and black pepper to the taste
- 1 yellow onion, chopped
- 2 garlic cloves, minced
- 3 zucchinis, grated

Directions:

1. In a bowl, mix zucchinis with garlic, onion, flour, salt, pepper, egg and dill, stir well, shape small patties out of this mix, spray them with cooking spray, place them in your air fryer's basket and cook at 370 degrees F for 6 minutes on each side.
2. Serve them as a snack right away.

Enjoy!

Nutrition: calories 60, fat 1, fiber 2, carbs 6, protein 2

Cauliflower Bars

Preparation time: 10 minutes **Cooking time:** 25 minutes

Servings: 12

Ingredients:

- 1 big cauliflower head, florets separated
- ½ cup mozzarella, shredded
- ¼ cup egg whites
- 1 teaspoon Italian seasoning
- Salt and black pepper to the taste

Directions:

1. Put cauliflower florets in your food processor, pulse well, spread on a lined baking sheet that fits your air fryer, introduce in the fryer and cook at 360 degrees F for 10 minutes.

2. Transfer cauliflower to a bowl, add salt, pepper, cheese, egg whites and Italian seasoning, stir really well, spread this into a rectangle pan that fits your air fryer, press well, introduce in the fryer and cook at 360 degrees F for 15 minutes more.

3. Cut into 12 bars, arrange them on a platter and serve as a snack

Enjoy!

Nutrition: calories 50, fat 1, fiber 2, carbs 3, protein 3

Pesto Crackers

Preparation time: 10 minutes **Cooking time:** 17 minutes

Servings: 6

Ingredients:

- ½ teaspoon baking powder
- Salt and black pepper to the taste
- 1 and ¼ cups flour
- ¼ teaspoon basil, dried
- 1 garlic clove, minced
- 2 tablespoons basil pesto
- 3 tablespoons butter

Directions:

1. In a bowl, mix salt, pepper, baking powder, flour, garlic, cayenne, basil, pesto and butter and stir until you obtain a dough.
2. Spread this dough on a lined baking sheet that fits your air fryer, introduce in the fryer at 325 degrees F and bake for 17 minutes.
3. Leave aside to cool down, cut crackers and serve them as a snack.

Enjoy!

Nutrition: calories 200, fat 20, fiber 1, carbs 4, protein 7

Pumpkin Muffins

Preparation time: 10 minutes **Cooking time:** 15 minutes
Servings: 18

Ingredients:

- ¼ cup butter
- ¾ cup pumpkin puree
- 2 tablespoons flaxseed meal
- ¼ cup flour
- ½ cup sugar
- ½ teaspoon nutmeg, ground
- 1 teaspoon cinnamon powder
- ½ teaspoon baking soda
- 1 egg
- ½ teaspoon baking powder

Directions:

1. In a bowl, mix butter with pumpkin puree and egg and blend well.
2. Add flaxseed meal, flour, sugar, baking soda, baking powder, nutmeg and cinnamon and stir well.

3. Spoon this into a muffin pan that fits your fryer introduce in the fryer at 350 degrees F and bake for 15 minutes.
4. Serve muffins cold as a snack.

Enjoy!

Nutrition: calories 50, fat 3, fiber 1, carbs 2, protein 2

Zucchini Chips

Preparation time: 10 minutes **Cooking time:** 1 hour **Servings:** 6

Ingredients:

- 3 zucchinis, thinly sliced
- Salt and black pepper to the taste
- 2 tablespoons olive oil
- 2 tablespoons balsamic vinegar

Directions:

1. In a bowl, mix oil with vinegar, salt and pepper and whisk well.
2. Add zucchini slices, toss to coat well, introduce in your air fryer and cook at 200 degrees F for 1 hour.
3. Serve zucchini chips cold as a snack.

Enjoy!

Nutrition: calories 40, fat 3, fiber 7, carbs 3, protein 7

Beef Jerky Snack

Preparation time: 2 hours **Cooking time:** 1 hour and 30 minutes

Servings: 6

Ingredients:

- 2 cups soy sauce
- ½ cup Worcestershire sauce
- 2 tablespoons black peppercorns
- 2 tablespoons black pepper
- 2 pounds beef round, sliced

Directions:

1. In a bowl, mix soy sauce with black peppercorns, black pepper and Worcestershire sauce and whisk well.
2. Add beef slices, toss to coat and leave aside in the fridge for 6 hours.
3. Introduce beef rounds in your air fryer and cook them at 370 degrees F for 1 hour and 30 minutes.
4. Transfer to a bowl and serve cold.

Enjoy!

Nutrition: calories 300, fat 12, fiber 4, carbs 3, protein 8

Honey Party Wings

Preparation time: 1 hour and 10 minutes **Cooking time:** 12 minutes **Servings:** 8

Ingredients:

- 16 chicken wings, halved
- 2 tablespoons soy sauce
- 2 tablespoons honey
- Salt and black pepper to the taste
- 2 tablespoons lime juice

Directions:

1. In a bowl, mix chicken wings with soy sauce, honey, salt, pepper and lime juice, toss well and keep in the fridge for 1 hour.
2. Transfer chicken wings to your air fryer and cook them at 360 degrees F for 12 minutes, flipping them halfway.
3. Arrange them on a platter and serve as an appetizer.

Enjoy!

Nutrition: calories 211, fat 4, fiber 7, carbs 14, protein 3

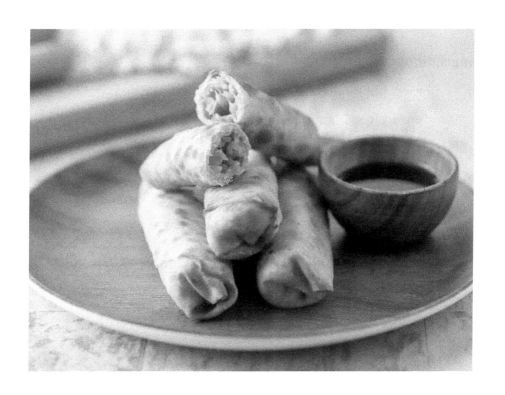

Salmon Party Patties

Preparation time: 10 minutes **Cooking time:** 22 minutes

Servings: 4

Ingredients:

- 3 big potatoes, boiled, drained and mashed
- 1 big salmon fillet, skinless, boneless
- 2 tablespoons parsley, chopped
- 2 tablespoon dill, chopped
- Salt and black pepper to the taste
- 1 egg
- 2 tablespoons bread crumbs
- Cooking spray

Directions:

1. Place salmon in your air fryer's basket and cook for 10 minutes at 360 degrees F.
2. Transfer salmon to a cutting board, cool it down, flake it and put it in a bowl.
3. Add mashed potatoes, salt, pepper, dill, parsley, egg and bread crumbs, stir well and shape 8 patties out of this mix.
4. Place salmon patties in your air fryer's basket, spry them with cooking oil, cook at 360 degrees F for 12 minutes, flipping them halfway, transfer them to a platter and serve as an appetizer.

Enjoy!

Nutrition: calories 231, fat 3, fiber 7, carbs 14, protein 4

Conclusion

Air frying is one of the most popular cooking methods these days and air fryers have become one of the most amazing tools in the kitchen.

Air fryers help you cook healthy and delicious meals in no time! You don't need to be an expert in the kitchen in order to cook special dishes for you and your loved ones!

You just have to own an air fryer and this great air fryer cookbook!

You will soon make the best dishes ever and you will impress everyone around you with your home cooked meals!

Just trust us! Get your hands on an air fryer and on this useful air fryer recipes collection and start your new cooking experience!

Have fun!

Lightning Source UK Ltd.
Milton Keynes UK
UKHW021846220221
379219UK00004B/596